————————Acclaim for Michelle Myers-Walters'
I Didn't Miscarry Her...She Died.————

"As a mother whose baby died at 8 weeks gestation, I was inspired by Michelle's ability to put into words what many women feel when going through this kind of grief. It is encouraging to know that other women have experienced the same loss and have grown to be stronger women through the process. This book will help many women struggling with the same ordeal know that they are not alone."
Dr. Kayci Lewis, D.O.

"This book will provide comfort to those who hurt, bring peace to those who mourn, and will help women find the courage to hold on until the dawn of renewed life. Through her first-hand account of the loss of her *angel* child Myers-Walters reaches the heart as only a mother could. For those who have recently lost an unborn child or those who continue to struggle...this book will speak peace to your soul and hope to your heart."
Dr. Chuck Edgington
Neuropsychologist

"Michelle captures the realness and despair that a women feels. However, she gives her readers the hope and validation that they so greatly need at that time in their lives. Michelle Myers-Walters captures a little bit of everyone's story in her own."
Ashley Thomas, M.S., CCC-SLP
Speech-Language Pathologist
Autism Advocate

I Didn't Miscarry Her... She Died

— A Mother's Perspective on Miscarriage and Loss —

Michelle L. Myers-Walters

ISBN 13: 978-0-9820141-6-5
ISBN 10: 0-9820144-6-3

Published in 2009 in the United States by
Adsum Press, a division of
Woolstrum Publishing House LLC.

www.adsumpress.com

Printed in the United States of America
on acid-free paper.
All trademarks are owned by
their respective companies.

16 15 14 13 12 11 10 09 08 07 06 05 04 03 02 01

Dedicated to...

Our angel baby, *Sarah Faith*
Thank you for letting me be your mommy.

And my friends:
Kimberly Casseday
Danna Davis (3 angels)
Misty Devine (*Mattie Aileen*)
Amanda Hollinger
Amy McCrabb (little angels)
Carolyn Hawkinson-Pruett (*Daniel & Aurora*)
Kim Sweeder
Jasmin Valentine (angel)
Elizabeth Walker (*Carlos*)
Sarah Weingartner (*Gwendolyn Paige*)
Wendy Young
Lori
Susie

Table of Contents

Miscarriage

Mis-car-riage
Function: *noun*;
Date: circa 1652
1: corrupt or incompetent management;
especially: failure in the administration
of justice

2: spontaneous expulsion of a
human fetus before it is viable
and especially between the
12th and 28th weeks of gestation

Definition from Merriam-Webster Dictionary

I wonder who the bright light bulb was that decided losing a baby should be synonymous with incompetent management. By definition alone, the word *miscarriage* blames the mother for her role in the death of her unborn child.

For years now, many of us have dealt with the term miscarriage, and it doesn't sit well with us that this definition exists. It should be changed. To what, I don't know. What about *uterine loss of life*, or *gestational death*? I haven't found a phrase that works for me just yet, but I think it is ignorant to assume 'miscarriage' is justifiable.

So why are you reading this book?

Have you been branded with the word *miscarriage*? Do you feel this weight of horror that makes you cry at the sound of newborns, and run from pregnant people? Or maybe you're a friend or loved one of someone who lost their baby and you're searching for a way to support them.

Whatever reason you picked up this book, know that it is full of conversation and information about losing a baby while pregnant. This book is written to empower those who are weary and enlighten some who are confused. This journey can be very confusing some times. Heck, I'm still confused, and it's been five years since *Sarah* left.

Medical terms that make no sense, insensitive doctors that want you to hurry up, and let's not forget to mention the friends and relatives that just don't seem to get what you're going through. Well, don't be upset at them. How can they be expected to understand, when we struggle to comprehend what has happened?

So, **I got tired of being silent and wrote this book.** I don't want to be ashamed when someone finds out about my miscarriage. It wasn't my fault. Herein lies words that will support, comfort and connect with you on this journey. A journey where as women, we define the experience of losing our children, and refuse to adhere to man's definition.

You didn't mis-carry or drop the ball.
You didn't mishandle your pregnancy...
your baby died.

1ST THING'S FIRST

Father asked us:
"what was God's noblest work."
Anna said men,
but I said babies.
Men are often bad,
but babies never are.

Louisa May Alcott

Ever since I was a little girl, I dreamed about the day that I would be able to become a mother.

Page 1

Even at a young age, I wrote down the names of future daughters or sons and believed it was one of the most special things that could happen to a girl.

I think it started the day my mother brought my little brother home from the hospital. I fondly remember the joy that surrounded the occasion, and I loved helping to take care of him. When I met the love of my life, I knew that he would be the father of my children.

Five pregnancies and six children later, (twins once) I found myself pregnant with our seventh child. I didn't really think about what could go wrong, even though I had experienced hypertension, pre-term labor, and gestational diabetes before. I took it for granted that *pregnancy* equaled a new baby in the family.

Our Angel Baby's name is *Sarah Faith*.

I wrote her name so many times, while she lay beneath my heart, and I couldn't wait to see it written on a birth certificate. She was to be born in the fall.

When Do You Celebrate Being Pregnant?

First Heartbeat...
First Trimester?

I remember the day I found out I was pregnant. It was the morning of my thirty-first birthday. As soon as I peed on the stick, I was so excited I could hardly hold the test in my hand. I didn't need to see an ultrasound picture, and a heartbeat wouldn't have been possible. The spirit of my child burned brightly in my soul, and warmth spread throughout me. I WAS SO EXCITED!

A brand new life within me has begun
There are no words,
when it comes to the young.
The sweetness that comes from the
smell of their skin,
The way they coo brings such joy within.

Oh, God, you have blessed me
more than you should.
I could never repay you, oh...that i could.
This gift you bestow so gentle and sweet,
Will forever be loved, my joy is complete.

That was in November, 2003. As time progressed, I had an unusual feeling that surfaced. I began to think something would be wrong with *Sarah*, and I hated that thought.

I remember praying around Christmas time, that if something horrible was going to be wrong with her, I'd rather that God take her now. I couldn't bear to see my child in physical pain.

A PRAYER SHOULD NEVER HAUNT YOU, BUT THAT ONE DID FOR THE NEXT FEW YEARS.

January 15th, I awoke in the middle of the night...

SCREAMING.

"Why Do I Feel So Alone?"

My husband kept trying to assure me that he was right there with me, but he misunderstood. I felt like something cold had ripped across my belly, and I knew that *Sarah's* spirit had left my body. The alone that I was talking about had nothing to do with who lay beside me. It was about who had grown inside of me.

The next morning the spotting started. I wanted to believe everything was fine, but this had never happened to me before. I knew in my heart it wasn't ok, but I kept trying to convince myself that it was nothing. As the day went on, I kept reassuring myself that it was nothing.

Finally, the next day, I knew the bleeding wasn't going to stop. My husband came and took me to the emergency room. I remember lying on the table as they did the ultrasound. The table was COLD and HARD, and I felt like a ton of weight lay on me. My heartbeat echoed inside my mind, and darkness rested on me. I didn't want to look at the screen, but it was like a magnet made me face toward the image.

Over the years I had seen many ultrasound screens. It was always a source of joy and anticipation, but now, it was a horrible view of a figure that I couldn't recognize. The image I saw on the screen wasn't shaped like it should have been, at ten weeks. It should have looked different. Worse than that, there was no sound.

How are you supposed to respond when someone tells you your baby didn't make it? I think they need to have some sort of protocol for dealing with these things in the emergency room. I've heard many horror stories that far exceed my own, but I was coldly told the baby wouldn't grow, and asked "Did I want to have a D&C" or let it naturally abort?

I Didn't Miscarry Her...She Died.

The word 'abort' snapped me out of my stupor, and I began to cry. That's another word you don't think about when planning to have children.

'Naturally abort' is also on my list of top hated phrases used in this process.

The Doctor Was Factual,

I Was A Mess.

I kept saying I felt pregnant, even though they told me I had a miscarriage. The ultrasound looked weird, and I couldn't grasp what they were saying. The bleeding got worse, and all things seemed to indicate that I had lost the baby. Once again, all the wording seemed to blame it on me.

I HAD LOST our child.

I've hated the word miscarriage from the first moment I heard it. It seemed to be a word that validated the unwarranted feelings of guilt and regret. Here I was already devastated by the fact that my baby had died inside of me. Now, I felt a label nailed to my forehead. A flashing sign that told everyone what I had done.

Even though there were people in my life who told me daily it was not my fault, something inside of me haunted the logical sides of my mind. The thought that I had done something wrong to lose her just wouldn't go away. I had to have done something wrong. It was my job to carry the baby and I HADN'T DONE MY JOB.

This is the reason
why mothers
are more devoted to their children
than fathers:
it is that they suffer more
in giving them birth
and are more certain
that they are their own.

———————

Aristotle

The weeks passed and I still *Felt* pregnant. I was told you could feel pregnant for awhile after having a miscarriage. Not only that, everyone was different, so there was no way to tell me how long the feeling would last.

No ultrasounds were ordered, and I felt miserable. I stayed in a dark room at first, unable to even stand the light. Doctor's said that I had developed depression or anxiety, so I was put on medication to calm me. The days were immeasurable, the moments torturous. I couldn't find my way out of the darkness of loss.

Every now and then, I would hear my other children's voices out in the hall. It was like this constant reminder of what would never be. No matter what I tried to think about to remove the gloominess, I remained in a world taunted by giggles.

How is this not my fault?

I was supposed to see
my baby **safely** through

to the other side.

I Didn't Miscarry Her...She Died.

No matter how many smiling faces I see
No matter how many times I hear, "mommy!"
There's one voice that seems to be missed,
There's one head I'll never kiss...

I feel like I'm broken and my chest won't breathe
I feel like someone hit me, I've fallen to my knees.
Desperate and sick, is it...to hold on?
Is there some time limit before I'll see the dawn?

Sarah in my sleep...**Sarah** in my head...
I'm so tired of crying...poor **Sarah** is dead.
I believe there is a God, and mercy I do need
How do I become thankful... When all I do is grieve?

I try to keep on smiling, inside everyone's unaware
I feel I'm slowing dying, sometimes. . .I don't care.
Sarah if you're listening, mommy loves you still,
I just want to hold you...to know that you were...real.

Everyone keeps telling me, how special I am blessed.
But sometimes deep inside of me....everything's a mess.
I love my children, shouldn't that be enough?
Am I just being selfish, or is losing #7 too much?

I felt her spirit leave me, from within me torn
I found myself awake screaming.
Maybe I was dreaming?
I feel like a walking nightmare, never to awake
God, can you please tell me, "Did I make some mistake?"

Everyone's moment is different.

No two stories are exactly the same, even if the two people witnessed the same event. The moment that you find out your baby is no longer inside of you is one you will never ever forget. It's not like the movies, where time slows down and you can see what's going to happen. Instead, it moved so fast, I couldn't catch my breath. I couldn't slow things down and hold on to reality.

Some people are told they have molar pregnancies. Some people are told they have a blighted ovum. Some people have a multiple pregnancy, lose one baby, and go on to carry its twin or other siblings to term. There are all sorts of terms and labels written on our medical charts.

Whatever gestational week you were on our stories may be different, but they all involve loss. That's one of the reasons I'm writing this book. Some women have been heartbroken when a seven week pregnancy ended. Can you believe some people think the shorter the pregnancy, the shorter your grief should be?

That line of thinking is absurd.

When a woman learns she is pregnant, we don't just plan the rest of the afternoon, we immediately plan the upcoming year.

Some people figure out how much maternity leave they will need from work. Some people think about how they will feel on the vacation that is planned for months away. I thought about what other child's birthday would be close to hers. I thought about how we would ensure that child a good birthday party, even if I went into labor.

Unlike me, some people wait until they are past the first trimester. I normally couldn't contain myself that long, and if I told my husband, the cat was definitely out of the bag.

But what happens when you lose a baby? You don't feel the overwhelming urge to get on the phone and call people. If you run into someone at the store, are you obligated to tell them? What happens when someone mentions the baby, and how happy they are that you are pregnant?

No one could be prepared for that. One of the hardest things was telling my children. My eldest at the time was almost ten, and she had been so excited when we had told them we were expecting. It was so hard to watch her accept the words, that the baby would not be born.

Expecting.

I guess that's one thing that makes it so devastating. We truly expect things to be fine. We truly expect for a baby to eventually arrive. It would be nuts for things to be any different. Most people don't find out they're pregnant and think of all the horrible things that could happen. Well, at least not before your first loss.

*Expectation is the root
of all heartache.*

William Shakespeare

DIDN'T KNOW

THAT

COULD HAPPEN

A single event can awaken within us a
stranger totally unknown to us.
To live is to be slowly born.

Antoine de Saint-Exupery

The crystal ball that predicts the future was absent. No one could have expected what happened next, least of all me.

Sixteen weeks gestation didn't seem like a date we would even recognize during this pregnancy. It appeared to have ended nine weeks earlier, and no one would listen to the crazy, grief stricken mother who said she still felt pregnant.

My eldest two daughters were dancing around, practicing for a dance recital, and I suddenly felt ill. Thinking that it was just something I ate, I ran to the bathroom. Overwhelmed by stomach cramps and pain, I hurried to undo my clothing.

Within minutes, I delivered the remains of my daughter, *Sarah*. Apparently her body had kept growing, and she looked approximately ten to twelve weeks. My choice to allow my body to naturally deal with losing *Sarah* had not gone ideally.

My mind disconnected from my body. I cleaned up the mess, walked back out, and went to my daughters' dance class. There were no thoughts; there wasn't anything. I guess it was shock. It was the reality of that horrible moment.

The next morning I awoke, completely out of it. I was rushed to the emergency room.

DIAGNOSIS. PANIC ATTACK.

I didn't miscarry anything...

my baby died.

Am I naive to think it would get easier with time?
Maybe that's just because everyone fed me that line.
Hold on to memories, hold on to time,
What kind of memories, does miscarriage leave behind?

I wish I had a doll, a dress she would have worn,
Maybe then I could smell it, and not feel so torn.
How can my heart be so full, and my arms be empty,
I'm tired of people telling me I have so plenty.

Plenty of what? Grief and despair?
Plenty of days, trying to care.
I'm clawing at sanity, a life I once knew
But without her I'm clueless...Does this happen to you?

I used to be so positive, outgoing and free.
That was before miss-carriage visited me.
And what is it to mis carry a child might I asked?
I held on so tight, but the pregnancy didn't last.

There is no expert reasoning, I'm sick of them all.
Only you here understand the echoes of the empty hall.
Back and forth between sleep and awake,
Did I hear a baby cry...No, my mistake.

So where do we find hope and courage
Why do we go on?
Does somebody have the magic answer?
Well, let's try this one on.

A mother...That's it, I think definition clear.
Grieving those we've lost, unconscious of the years.
Miscarriage, yeah whatever, as a mom here's the word...
"Death of a child" seems more adequate,
but some have never heard.

If one more single person asks, "why are you so sad,
Your baby wasn't even born, never even had?"
I'd take an amniotic sac, and smack
them in the head,
Then ask them, "now, how do you feel,
Was that hit fake...Or was it real?"

I want to go to the highest mountain
And shout out loud her name...
Sarah Faith was my seventh child
That fact will never change.

Does anybody understand how bad I hurt inside?

Un-being dead isn't being ALIVE.

e. e. cummings

Clinging to the bathroom wall a day later, I slid down the cold tile crying. I couldn't stand to think about what had happened. I don't know how long I lay with my face pressed against the floor, but I remember sobbing even when the tears dried up.

The loneliness of that moment is unbearable to think about, even now. I felt lost, and no thoughts made any sense. The sound of my other children laughing made me crazy. It was like they were imaginary and disconnected from me. I wanted to take care of them and be my old self, but I wasn't. I didn't know how to find that person in this moment.

Shattered isn't a word reflected in my mind
It's so much more than that, it's
contemplating mankind.
The meaning of life, I don't know if I can try,
Some say it is purpose, but mine just died.

That's how I feel whether it's right or wrong,
I don't care anymore…my heart is now gone.
If it could beat, I know I couldn't stand the pain,
It would confirm that I'm alive…again and again.

God let me cease thoughts and just cry
Maybe then it would be easier as I slowly die.
It would be less dramatic, more clear and defined,
Just let me drift away from my mind.

Ripped away from the warmth of innocence
Now I'm running toward the darkness.
I should run away, but I don't know how.
There's only the knowledge that is too profound.

I stood looking in the mirror, horrified by my reflection. My belly still looked like it housed a baby, but I knew it was empty. I was still feeling sick to my stomach this morning, and my breasts felt like they had gone through a wringer.

I needed someone who would understand. Looking around my immediate family, I didn't know anyone who I felt could truly understand. I went online to a miscarriage message board, and found a group of women who understood my pain.

They had similar experiences, and knew the heartache that accompanied this type of loss. No matter what gestation, we all understood the unspoken about miscarriages.

Many people posted poems or prose, others just wrote letters back and forth. I was fortunate enough to make some friends that are still in my life years later.

As I Sit And Listen, And Read All The Post
I Feel Haunted And Hollow...As If A Ghost.
A Shadow Of The Woman I Used To Be,
Ever Since I Lost The Child That Grew Within Me.

One Moment I'm Screaming, One Moment I Cry
One Moment She Was Living...The Next She Died.
God, I'm Just Drowning In So Much Despair
But Somehow I Keep Going, Somehow I Care.

But Why, When I Took Such Good Care Of Myself?
Why? When I Put Pregnancy Above Everything Else?
I Wish I Had Someone To Hit Or To Blame,
But I Look To Myself Again And Again.

Logically, I Know, The Hormones And Such
Caused Her To Leave, For Us To Lose Touch...
But If There Were Something Easier To Name
I Could Pin Point A Moment And Say,
"Ah, There's The Blame."

But There's Not, And I'm Left Thinking Things,
Things That Only A Mother's Ache Sings...
My Beautiful Child I Thought To Hold In My Hands,
Has Gone Away To A Far Away Land.

I'd Bargain With God, But What Could I Give?
I Have Nothing Of Value, Except That I Live.
If For No Other Reason, To Make Known For Sure,
That Babies Are Precious, Not To Be Ignored.

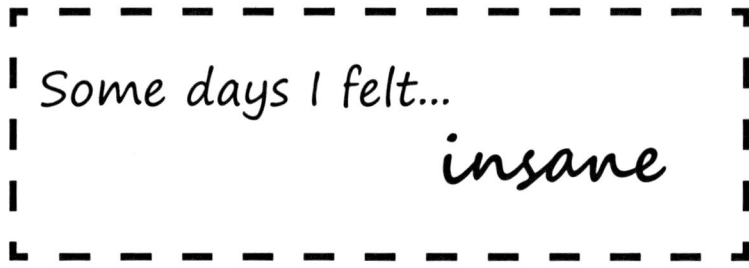

Some days I felt... *insane*

The early days were the hardest. I was torn between enjoying the children that ran around the house, and grieving the one that was lost. Some of my "Christian" (and I use the word loosely) friends, would point out that at least I had children.

My response was always the same.

It focused around the verse in the Bible, about the shepherd leaving the ninety-nine sheep to find the **one**.

Then Jesus told them this parable:

Suppose one of you has a hundred sheep
And loses one of them. Does he not leave
the ninety-nine in the open country
and go after the lost sheep
until he finds it?

Luke 15:3-4

One sheep meant just as much
as the others that were safe.

Now I know that the previous verse deals with the
salvation of mankind, but it comforted me somehow,
reminding me that it was ok to be upset.

My angel baby, *Sarah*, meant just as much to me,
as the children that I was blessed to have
running around at my feet.

Sometimes I imagine she's here with me....

Was that a giggle, was that a laugh?
It must just be the wind.
Did someone say, "mommy?" Did someone need me?
It must just be the wind.

A warm sensation that begins in my mind,
And sweeps over my whole body in time.
Is it my imagination, or something i really felt?
It must just be the wind.

I imagine she's playing peek-a-boo
And hiding behind a tree.
If i could just turn around quick enough,
Little feet running i'd see.

Sarah, my voice calls loud
Sarah, echoes throughout a crowd.
And if i shut my eyes i swear
I hear her answer, "mommy, i'm here."

I cried a lot, but hey,
if Jesus could cry...

Jesus wept.
John 11:35

why not me?

When the tears stopped falling as quickly, I tried to find other ways to express my grief. I must have cleaned and re-cleaned things a million times. By this time, my anxiety was terrible. I could hardly get myself to move or act normal. When I wanted to sleep, I couldn't, when I should have been awake, I slept.

Doctors seemed to be experimenting with my medication. Some things would make me loopy, while others would make me completely freak out. One medication made the light hurt my eyes, and I felt like I was constantly on the verge of vomiting. I knew everyone was trying to help me feel better, but at times it backfired.

I was so thankful that *my mother* was around during this time. She took care of my children, cooked and cleaned. I tried to do what I could, but I failed miserably at trying to act human. It was as if I wasn't in my body anymore. An alien life form of grief moved in and took over my thoughts.

Now I know tons of people who say they've been through a tragedy, and somehow found the strength to go on as usual. I'm not a hater, I think that's amazing. I wasn't one of those people, and chances are, if you're reading this book...you aren't either.

Maybe it has to do with environment, culture, or simply personality. I don't know, but I was very moved by the loss of my child. Losing *Sarah* is one of the most defining moments of my life. I'm still figuring out some things about myself because of this.

Soaring far into the heavens...
A beautiful cocoon, within it grows the graceful butterfly...
Pulsing life I can feel when I rest my hand
upon my womb...
And suddenly, you are gone
And suddenly, I am no longer more than one.

I'll never see you soar, or dance in the sunlight of this world.
The wings you have now are more than
I would have given...
I keep falling off the mountain, is it you that
keeps catching me?
I keep falling...I keep drowning...
Thoughts of you keep touching me....

I look up into the blinding light of the sun
I wonder where my strength comes from.
Because i am so weak...I am crippled by my grief
Used to sit and cry...Now my eyes are dry.

Questions, questions flying around and hitting me,
There are no answers, there is no destiny.
Beautiful butterfly, are you soaring now
Where angels dance....Do you wear a crown?

My sweet, sweet princess...**Sarah**

No doubt exists that all women are CRAZY;
it's only a question of degree.

W. C. Fields

MULTIPLE
PERSONALITY
PLANET

I started living in this world of chaos.

I Didn't Miscarry Her...She Died.

A world where I had to always be *two* people at once,
equally functioning at the same time.

On one hand,
I was wounded and bleeding—on the other, I was the
happy mother, taking care or her brood and
making her home happy.

My body was like this GIANT PUPPET,
and something was pulling the strings.

Always a mother, always my sweet child...
But you have to believe, that somewhere
A little angel hovers over...always near.
To comfort you this month with whispers of hope
Never give up? We try...just to cope.

We wear 2 faces, one for the crowd
the other cries tears, and screams within, loud!
Oh, to be free from the sad memories,
But longing to remember, is sometimes the worse of these.

Anniversary moments, anniversary days
I'm so sick of waiting for them to pass or to fade.
But I don't think they do, or that they will
But we have to find solace, and peace somewhere still.

So I try to find moments to remember the feel.
To remember the warmth of my smile, knowing she was real.
And even though I can't remember her move...
I know she's here hovering...hovering still.

Pregnant people drove me nuts.

Seeing a pregnant person during the month of August was hard. Not to mention, when people had a child around the same time.

It's not something I sat around doing on purpose; it was just this weird morphed world of torture.

Every newborn was like a giant dagger that pierced the wound in my heart.

Before all this had happened, I was the first person to go nuts making stuff for other people's babies. As soon as friends or family said they were expecting, I lovingly and excitedly crocheted blankets, hats and sweaters.

After, well, I ran from pregnant people. *Literally*! I could be in the store and see someone pregnant and go out of my way to avoid them. And because I had so many little children at the time, people would stop me and ask me questions in the baby section. I absolutely hated getting diapers in Wal-mart.

Once, a woman saw me in the sewing department with the children. She said, "Oh, God, I hear you're having another one." She didn't say it nice at all. Of course, she had no idea I had lost a baby. So I replied, rather loudly,

"No, actually, she just died."

The look on the fellow shopper's faces was stunned. The woman just about swallowed her tongue, but I managed to hold my face perfectly as I walked off with my toddlers in tow.

I'm not sure when it happened, but as time passed, I wasn't as sensitive to comments like that. I must have cried for two days over that incident. Now, I look back, and I learned some very valuable lessons.

1. *I don't owe anyone an explanation.*
2. *Some people don't recognize that children are a blessing.*

My large family bothered her for some reason, but I would have given anything to restore the child I had just lost.

My husband, wonderful man that he is, tried to console me best he could. But every word of comfort he directed my way seemed to annoy me because I knew he couldn't really understand. He could never fully experience the resonating joy that expounds when you feel a first movement or realize another soul is housed within you.

I found such salvation from my friends on the message board. Some of us decided to break off into our own little group. We formed strong friendships as the years passed, and I knew I wasn't alone in my struggle.

Through the warmth of friendship, I was reminded of the comforting love of God. Even though I felt abandoned by all that I knew optimistic, I was led to loving women who helped me see the love of God within.

All we can do is decide to take
each step day by day.

I got so tired of all the diagnoses of what could be
wrong, I had lost my baby. I couldn't focus
on the present, because a part of me
was stuck back in that day.

The day I felt myself split and
become someone else.

It requires more courage to suffer than to die.
Napoleon Bonaparte

Becoming this new person hasn't been easy. When I was a little girl, dreaming about being a mommy, I didn't figure in the equation a baby not being born.

And just like people adopt children who are not born from their physical bodies, even though my child was never "born," I don't love her any less.

Today may a warmth of peace, caress the tears upon your cheek.
Today may you find comfort, wherever you may seek.
The anguish in your heart will never fade,
but you will find courage to face it more, with the passing of days.

A sweet Angel will be with you, you are now never alone.
Because when a child passes, their spirit is felt within your own.
There are no words to take away, the pain you will always bare...
But we are here to support you, with so much love to share.

No words can ever convey
the deepness of the sorrow that has come your way.
Dream of soft kisses upon your head
left by an angel baby instead.

There is no comfort, no "thing" that will fix
all of the hurt, so much...you are sick.
But believe you are alive to hope and dream,
feel the baby's spirit, as faint as it may seem.

Doesn't matter if nobody else knew,
you and your husband are dealing with what is true.
You have lost your little, lovely sweet one,
when their frail life, had just begun.

I hope you find some comfort here
where others in your hurting share.
With all my heart, I say to yours
Just get through each day after the one before.

I Didn't Miscarry Her...She Died.

It began to amaze me, how many women have experienced this type of loss. When I finally had the courage to say

'I've lost a baby,'

I was stunned to hear a relative or friend talk about their own or someone they knew.

If it's such a common denominator in so many women's lives, why is it such a guilty thing to talk about? Sometimes, it was almost shameful, as if I had made the ultimate mistake in life. I allowed my child not to make it. Sounds crazy I know, but the overwhelming grief wasn't accompanied with rational thought all the time.

_____

When people ask how many children I have

_____ ...I stumble.

We've all had that moment. The moment someone asks how many children you have. I hate that question. Seems awful innocent, but it's like this giant set up of pain, designed to torture a woman who's had a loss like this.

In the early days, I would almost choke and end up crying within minutes. After a year or two, it was still the weirdest thing to answer. It's only now, about five years later, that I have finally found an answer that sits well with me.

Depending on the questioner, I will say the current number, or I will say a number and one *angel baby*. Most people end the questioning, either way, and I've gotten over feeling obligated to answer further.

What's been really eye-opening is to hear other people respond, when I mention *Sarah* as an angel baby. I can't even count the times other women have said they lost a child from the womb. **Perfect strangers instantly feel connected, knowing that someone understands the journey they are on.**

It doesn't end, but it changes as the days and weeks pass. I will always miss the undeniable feeling that I know I felt from *Sarah*. But I'm learning how to appreciate my time with her, as brief as it was, and know that I will see her again.

We are all connected by a thin thread,
a line of commonality, layers of sorrow shed.
Know that every tear you cry,
you cry for me when mine are too dry.

And every smile you make,
opposes the sound of my heartbreak.
Together we all here will remain strong,
When you are weak, I will open my arms.

Open wounds upon our soul,
I expect our babies' spirits will know.
Their mommies loved them more than life
And they understand, why we weep this night.

All I can send you besides this (((hug)))
is the knowledge that though unknown by sight,
you are loved.
As the women of this thread of pain,
you have helped me find my strength, again...
and again.

Time passes so slowly...then all of a sudden, it's over.
The tears I cry now are different,
than the tears before.

Another baby?

As time passed, I learned to balance the two faces better and better. I think I began to fool myself a bit. By this time, I was pregnant again, but unlike any pregnancy I had ever had...

I Didn't Miscarry Her...She Died.

I felt nothing about this baby.

I had no idea how to connect with the pregnancy.

Sadness overwhelmed me instead of joy,

and I had thought another baby would restore **hope** and somehow save me from my sorrow. Instead, I felt guilty, when I felt happy about the new baby. In so many ways, it was a betrayal of *Sarah*.

I couldn't make sense of things.

Know little one, that mommy never forgets
I've got a memory that is more than mere thought.
It holds emotions and feelings,
of the short time you were here,
I'm sorry you left....my sweet, sweet dear...

My arms feel so empty, my heart is so full
of hopes and dreams, but where are you?
The center of my desires, the thing that drives,
can be found in the midst of the tears in my eyes.

Torn into pieces...you were torn from me
Sometimes I feel help-less, there's no reason I see.
But a mother is more than mere words that take place.
I'm an entity of love that transcends time...and space.

So I open my soul, and expose to all who read.
I give away my privacy and anonymity.
For the children that we've loss, for the hurt we bare
when you are slipping into sorrow,
reach out...we are here.

A glitter of hope, the future remains
and even though nothing from this point
will ever be the same.
A mother wears proud the scars of our journey...
We can never exactly know...
but we recognize the yearning.

So I'm pregnant again _____

It wasn't that I wasn't happy about it, but it wasn't like before. I went to sleep one night, exhausted from crying and trying to be ok.

I dreamed of a beautiful field of grass that lay beautifully beside a still, glistening, dark body of water.

Suddenly, a friend of mine named David that had passed on, was standing beside a tiny little girl. She was sitting on the grass with her back toward me, picking the petals off of yellow flowers. I figured she was around two years of age, and she reminded me of my other daughters, but I couldn't see her face.

As I neared them, David smiled at me nodding, and the little girl began to hum the song 'You Are My Sunshine.' I began to cry in my dream, and David let me know it was true. It was *Sarah* telling me that I was pregnant and going to have another daughter. Her name would be Sunshine.

When I woke up, I was the happiest I had been in a long time. Not only had I believed I saw *Sarah*, she had told me the baby I carried would be a girl. I jumped out of bed and ran to tell my husband. It was in the middle of the afternoon, and normally I was asleep from medication and exhaustion. Now, I was wide awake and out of my mind with joy.

My husband has always supported the 'feelings' that I've had over the years. I know with all my heart, God gave me that dream and I believed we were having a baby daughter. I wanted to be happy all the time about it. I thought I would smile for days...BUT THE JOY DIDN'T LAST.

Try as I might, the sorrow waved in and out of my mind. The nearer my approaching due date blazed on the calendar, the more panic entered my mind.

_____ *I don't want to forget my other baby.*

I tried to remember the moments that I was pregnant with *Sarah*. Somehow this new baby seemed to be making my memory blurred. It was a very confusing place to find myself living through, but I tried to be happy.

People around me kept commenting on how blessed we were to be having another baby, and don't get me wrong, I wanted to believe that. But it was what it was...

I was grieving the loss of one child,
while trying to celebrate the existence of a new one.

How can I grieve AND be happy?

Happiness is

beneficial

for the **BODY**,

But it is grief

that develops

the powers of

the mind.

———————

Marcel Proust

Ultimately, that's the answer to being human. Somehow we can go through the unimaginable, and still find the courage to go on and live productive lives.

There were some months that I felt so alone and abandoned by my beliefs. I hated to hear people talk about God never leaving or forsaking me. *I sincerely felt forsaken*, if not by God, by my own existence while my child was dead.

Most people misunderstand when a mother who's lost a child says that. Children aren't designed to pass on to Paradise before us. I hadn't even thought about that being a possibility, until *Sarah* left. Who sits up thinking about which one of their children might die before them? I'm sure there are people who plan their funerals and buy burial plots early, but I don't know of anyone who does that for their children.

So doesn't it go without saying,
a person might be a little nuts
when something like this happens?

Can people imagine what it's like to go from extreme joy, to extreme me sadness in the blink of an eye?

I was so happy the day I found out...

I remember the moment I thought I'd buy a pregnancy test.
My fingers flipped past boxes, until I found the
one that was the best.
First Response deemed to be my choice from the shelf,
felt great as I touched it, right now, there was nothing else.

Should I wait till the morning, or should I test now…?
Well, it says the first pee would better tell.
So I go to sleep happy, like a kid again with a smile
I would find out if I had a secret, in just a little while.

Is it morning, yes! The crack of dawn,
I've held all my pee all night long.
I run to the bathroom and tear down my clothes
now do I just pee on it, where did those directions go?

Ah, yes, the little strip thing is wet,
dare I wait the three minutes…ok, won't look yet.
Curiosity gets me and 1 minute in
Oh My God, is it pink…yes, again and again!!!

I don't know if I should scream or call my mom,
should I tell my dear husband, man! What a BOMB!!
I wonder if she will look like me,
maybe it's a boy, oh well, I can't wait to see.

A few weeks have passed, is that a spot I see?
No…No….it can't possibly be.
Ok, don't panic…sometimes people bleed,
I'll go to the hospital so they can reassure me.

I'm cramping a little, but hey, that's ok
It's probably just stretching…isn't that what they say?
I have great anticipation, when they say, "ultrasound."
I can't wait to see what is there, what they've found.

I Didn't Miscarry Her...She Died.

The story was so supposed to be so simple.

You get pregnant,

you enjoy your pregnancy to its fullest,

and then you have this wonderful baby.

The beginning of the poem above, truly expressed how happy I was at that moment. Every pregnancy moment gives me that utter sense of ultimate joy.

Isn't it crazy sometimes how you feel you might need to apologize for that? I'm generally a happy person, but while pregnant, it seemed that the sun shone even brighter. Even when pregnancies were difficult or I had to be on bed rest, joy was so apparent and abundant.

How can a person go from so much happiness to so much sorrow, without it affecting them in a very profound manner? I look back now and realize that I was too hard on myself. I thought there should have been a way for me to get through this better. Maybe I could have been less hysterical, or resisted the anxiety that consumed me.

My baby is gone, but even though I knew
the thoughts came too fast...I didn't know what to do!
Sometimes I'm screaming, I'm angry, insane...
Others times I'm weeping...and nothing remains.

Faith, what is that...I'll try to hold on
But my faith in living is somehow stripped...gone.
Was it my fault, did I do something wrong
Answer me, please, I'm broken...not strong.

I understand the two faces you wear today.
One is grieving...one refuses to give hope away.
But I believe we can hang on, and somehow be both
the grieving mother, and a new baby's host.

It doesn't take away the pain from the death
but a new baby growing...yes...you do feel blessed.
Somehow it proves to you, life goes on,
and until that happens, it's hard...but be strong.

TORNADO OF HELL

Where is God?

To
    believe
        in
            GOD
        is
        impossible;
    not
to
    believe
        in
            Him
                is
        ABSURD. _____
                    Voltaire

This chapter had to be written because I began to question my faith. At that time, I couldn't have acknowledged God any more than I could accept my baby had died. For weeks I couldn't wrap my head clearly around it.

Yes, I know some people rise above their human tendencies, find their faith strong and know that God is with them. And even though I logically knew that to be true, I flat out had this question floating around for weeks?

If God was as powerful as I knew Him to be, didn't he have the power to make my baby live?

And, even though I knew she was gone, I'd have moments I would imagine a miracle could happen, and I could wake up and she'd be back.

Now I'm not saying it was a rational thought—I wasn't in a rational state of mind.

Because I couldn't figure out how something so bad could happen, I began to think maybe He was angry at me.

What if I had finally done something so terrible, that He had taken my child away from me?

You place your hand upon an empty womb...
nothing you feel.
You place your hand upon your heart and it beats...
is it real?
Who placed your womb to grow beneath your heart?
And why would the same creator allow pain
when they are torn apart?

You were created beneath your mother's heart.
God allowed you to grow there right from the start.
So why allow your baby to die and leave you alone
Why not allow your womb to be its home?

Some things will be a mystery until the day we die.
But that doesn't erase the tears you now cry.
You may never know the answer to "why?"
But God sees every tear and hears every sigh.

For every stripe he bore on his back
tore at his flesh with the whip and its crack.
But He did it for love that He has for you
you question it now, but hold on to what is true.

Numb to feeling...I know and understand.
Losing the baby wasn't part of the plan.
But living in this world in these bodies of flesh
sometimes things go wrong, and
we're left in this mess.

When we were created, and then Jesus died
He promised to never leave,
to always be by your side.
So lean toward him, even if you're mad
He tells us to be angry...He allows us to be sad.

You are not unworthy, or worthless or wrong.
You're hurting inside, for your baby is gone.
But gone to this world, just means far away,
you will hold precious Angel babies someday.

Take the time you need to grieve and to miss
you are a mother...who's unfortunately on this list.
It wasn't your fault, you did nothing wrong,
Please, believe just enough, to keep holding on.

_____ Somehow you learn
to just be.
You live within
the sorrow and joy. _____

I wanted to wake up and things were as they were supposed to be. In my book, *Sarah* would be getting ready to be born. I would be decorating a crib with various blankets and taking photos. I wasn't supposed to be four months pregnant with this new baby. And even though I was happy she was growing well within me, I couldn't figure out how to feel at any given moment.

My head was one place, my heart was another. Or maybe, my heart had finally realized it could be split down the middle and still beat.

There's a piece of my heart in a faraway place
I wish I could put it back, because it can't be replaced.
Every time I breathe I feel it in my chest.
Every time I sigh, my whole body feels a mess.

It used to hurt so bad every time I took a breath,
but now as the days have gone by... I feel pain less and less.
But sometimes I'd rather feel pain than nothing at all.
Sometimes I'm just here...somehow I don't fall.

But I keep going on and living each day,
my heart seems so crippled, with that piece torn away.
People keep saying kind words as the day goes
But I hardly hear what they say, they don't even know.

The same simple sayings, the same stupid stares,
I'm falling to pieces...doesn't somebody realize it here!
I'm choking on memories and things I wanted to share
with a baby that's gone, that will never be here.

I'm angry, I'm sad... I'm just worn out now.
How can I find myself...God, I don't know how.
I look in a Bible, I find inspirational books
but none of them replace, my baby that was took.

A hole in my heart, I wish it were me...
I'd rather be gone...than without them here with me.
But I live to be living, I walk around still
Somehow I've lost the sparkle that made me feel.

Will it always be this way? Will I always cry each day?
Other people have children, they don't want anyway.
And here I sit, empty womb in my lap,
When I see tiny babies, I feel like I'm slapped.

Yes, I'm normally happy go lucky and free
But I've lost the baby that grew in me.
The only hope, I have that remains...
This hole in my heart...one day...will be changed.

The day that the child I lost lies on my chest.
And welcomes me home, to the place where she rest.
The Angels of mercy and Angels of Love
will spread wings around us, as we embrace...our first
hug.

I Didn't Miscarry Her...She Died.

I tried to think of my child being in a better place, but
what better place could there be,
than *within my arms?*

Sure, it was presumptuous for me to think
I knew better than God, but I am only human.
It's hard to see past today to the everlasting.

Could I love this baby as much as I would have loved her?

It wasn't supposed to be some type of competition. It wasn't supposed to be a balancing act with an invisible child and one that was to be born. I sat through the opening of baby presents and the joyful accolades with **guilt**. I wanted to smile, I wanted to sing, but how could I be so selfish with joy, when I couldn't even bury my last child.

And isn't that something that keeps you awake at night? For some of us there is no grave to visit. For others, they have the arduous task of up keeping a small place of internment. In some ways, maybe it's easier for me... without the grave.

As weird as it sounds, I would worry if the snow fell too heavy. I would worry about her being alone. As the holidays and birthdays passed, I would feel the undeniable pull to pay tribute in the place where her name was written on stone.

Then again...I had nothing from my pregnancy with **Sarah**.

I have nothing tangible to remind me of my baby.

That was definitely something that hurt the most. There was no physical evidence left of my loss with the baby. I had started a blanket the first month I found out I was pregnant, but in a moment of "tripping out," I gave it away to a lady walking on the street with her baby. Her child didn't even have a little coat on, so at the time, I figured the blanket was better in use than sitting on a shelf somewhere. I felt so selfish weeks later, when I cried thinking about the departure of that blanket. It was the only thing I had that made *Sarah* real.

A wonderful friend of mine, upon hearing my distress about the blanket, filled a beautiful box with things for my lost child. She even had *Sarah's* name monogrammed on a t-shirt and blanket, and it was such a beautiful acknowledgement of a life. I still have the box in my living room high on a shelf. Every once in a while, I will open it and run my fingers across the blanket and other cherished things. It doesn't bring sadness, it brings validation.

No picture of her, no memory of a smile...

Sometimes it almost seems crazy to miss a person I knew for such a short period of time. I used to think it would be easier not to remember her at all, but that goes against every instinct that is within my body. As time progressed, I began to realize it was ok to sit and think about her.

I learned that it was ok to remember the happy moments of that pregnancy. They were real, and they deserved to be acknowledged. So I decided to do two things at once.

1. I would acknowledge my current pregnancy.

2. And remember the happiness of finding out the previous baby was growing within me.

It wasn't as hard as I expected, it was more about realizing I didn't need permission to do both at the same time.

I Didn't Miscarry Her...She Died.

Remember the moment your face felt flush?
You had an idea...but you told yourself to hush?
The stir in your heart perhaps the idea was true,
that you might be pregnant...do you remember,
I do. (Smile)

> You envision of a glimpse of the possible moment,
> you'll walk up to DH, and say, "Hey, you've done it!"
> His face is so proud as he gives of a smile,
> and you both have a secret, you keep quiet,
> for awhile.

But soon, due to puking and all the gross stuff
you turn to your relatives and say, "Enough's enough!
We're having a baby, don't know when it's due
But we're blessed with another child,
and now, so are you!"

> Oh the shopping, the planning, the colors won't tell,
> will we find out this time, yeah...might as well!
> The new crib the old one, which one will we use?
> The pink or the blue one...GREEN! How can we lose!
> (Smile)

You roll over one day to flick something off your side,
Hey, there's nothing on me...the baby kicked INSIDE!
Then everyone you know has touched your belly,
Santa has nothing on you, this is some serious jelly!

The Holidays pass, as the due date gets near,
Anticipation, exhaustion...and sometimes fear....
Round as a basketball, full as Thanksgiving,
You begin to think, man, I hope my cervix is thinning.
(LOL)

And all of a sudden, you're off with a dash
to try to do it natural...maybe in a bath?
Forget it, the pain is just too much to bear,
Hey, doc! You got an epidural in here?!!!!!

Then suddenly you hear, "Hold on, it is crowning!"
You want to say, "Shut up! I know!
The pain's been mounting!"
With tons of pressure and a hesitant push,
out comes a slippery baby... in the buff. (LOL)

The smell of its hair, its soft batting eyes
you see yourself smiling, from the reflection inside.
And all of the pain, and fear that you had
was worth every moment...even the sad.

Why is it worth it, why did all of this start,
Because of the sound you hear now,
lying beneath your heart
And even though sadness, from the loss will be there,
There's nothing like stroking your cheek...across soft baby
hair. (Smile)

If time heals all...

then I need to get my watch fixed.

It wasn't something that happened overnight, but as time went on, I found it easier to breathe. The weight on my chest seemed lighter. I constantly read verses about giving your burden to the Lord to carry for you, but my logical, human side argued with that.

He couldn't understand this. He has never carried a baby inside of himself, so how could he understand this exact pain?

Was it possible, that He could understand the torment that I endured being a mere human?

And even if He could, would it matter to know He understood?

I would look at my Bible and refuse to open it some days. Other days, I literally rewrote Bible verses and tacked them above the headboard of my bed to sleep. I was living in a world caught between my mind and my spirit.

My logic dictated questions, my spirit sought the peace that comes in not knowing a specific answer. It sought the secret that we all long for in crisis; to truly know the presence of something bigger than us.

It's falling down on the altar of my pride,
sacrificing my impatience to the hands of time.
Trying to find a shadow on the wall,
even when it's so dark, and I'm blind.

And all the while voices keep ringing,
"Hey, stay positive, it will work out."
No matter how many times I smile, "ok,"
I want to just freak out and shout!!!!

What...I don't exactly know,
just seems like screaming is fun.
Of course I have hope or I wouldn't be here.
Sorry, some comments just seem dumb.

Blah, blah, blah, yeah, I know,
but the hour glass is going soooooooo slooooooooow.
Tears, sighs, laugh, which is which?
Sometimes I don't even know, and I act like a Witch. (Lol)

But I'm happy when I'm sad,
and angry when I smile.
Some people call me a little crazy,
guess I'll figure it all out after awhile.

So today I'll just stay positive,
whatever that is, what a laugh.
But, there's nothing else to do that makes sense,
Just wait.....for time.....to.....pass..........

As dumb as it sounds, I still found myself thinking I had done something wrong. Maybe it was the vitamins? Maybe it was the extra work I did? Maybe it was too soon after the twins were born? Maybe I had done something wrong, and this was God's way of punishing me?

Sure, the last question seems extreme to some, but I've come across many women whose faith made them ask this question. No matter what the denomination, there are many elements that make one feel good things are from God, bad things are from the Devil. If you're not living the way God wants you to, somehow bad things happen.

Well, that's not exactly what I found in the Bible.

And we know that in all things God
works for the good of those who love him,
Who have been called according
to his purpose.
Romans 8:28

P.S. I hated hearing this verse.

Ok, so if God was working good things out for me, how in the world would losing my baby fall beneath that category? I couldn't accept this verse, or what I thought it meant at the time. I thought it meant God would keep bad things like this from happening.

What I learned?

WHEN BAD THINGS HAPPEN,
GOD HAS A WAY OF MAKING GOOD THINGS
HAPPEN DESPITE THEM.

If being a Christian meant nothing bad happened, I'm sure it would be the leading belief in the world. Can you imagine NOTHING bad ever happening? It wouldn't make sense. Sometimes, things just go wrong. Many of us don't even know the reason we lost our babies. Some people get extensive testing, and have found answers that they always sought, and whatever someone feels like they need to do, I think they should do.

Ultimately though, the end result is the same for us all. We miss the children we lost from our womb. One good thing that has come despite that: I have found a connection with people that would have never happened except *Sarah* died.

Another: well, it's learning more about the God I say I believe in, and it led me on a journey to find out what I truly believed. So many times, people believe something because someone else did while they were children. *Now, I've learned so many things about the God I love that I don't believe I would have experienced if I had not been so broken and looking for peace.*

I've learned the beauty of compassion from a stranger,
and found the solidarity of women
who care about each other.

I've learned to do things for other babies
that I will never be able to do for her.
For every blanket that I will not crochet for *Sarah*,
I will give one to a baby in need,
which otherwise may not have one.
A small token by many measures,
but a gift from the heart nonetheless.

I am more blessed than I could ever deserve; to see the joy in a mother's eyes that I would have never met...if not for losing *Sarah*.

Love abounds where sorrow once lived,
and I believe I cherish life all the more,
for knowing death in such a manner.

You are not alone,
sadly many walk this road.
But our loving arms surround you,
to help you carry this load.
And even though our faith and
care cannot a life return,
as mothers of angel babies now,
we extend our care and concern.

The days seem endless, full of tears,
and grief so deeply sown.
Moments of light and laughter drift over,
and sadness becomes so known.
Though understanding evades you now,
no explanation clear,
Please know that although I can't offer much,
as kindred, I'll listen and hear.

Hope seems distant and far sometimes,
our spirits are crushed and bruised.
But Faith that things must get better,
we must strive to never lose.
The open wound upon your soul,
the seizure of your heart,
prevents your life from being the same;
so much has been torn apart.

But day to day you'll go on somehow,
to grieve, to live and believe.
Your Angel Babies watch over you,
their memory never to leave.
For even though within your womb,
their time on earth was not long;
your mother's love extends to them,
to clouds and far beyond.

WADE THROUGH THE WATER OR GRAB THE ROPE

*A woman is like a tea bag—
you can't tell how strong she is
until you put her in hot water.*
_____
Nancy Reagan

Each day I breathe...I still feel pain,
but I breathe and think of my sweet child again.
And though I'll never hold her, or gently touch her face,
I thank the Lord, but for one moment's grace.

Grace to see the sun still rise.
Even though some days, it's through tears that I cry.
Grace to kiss the people I love,
and look forward to see the baby...that lives far above.

Thankfulness means many different things now;
somehow I make it...even though I wonder how.
I know there's a light that blinds through this dark sea,
and one day a little girl's face will comfort me.

So each day I breathe, I try not to hold my breath.
I ask the Lord, "Please, take care of the rest..."
After all I've gone through, my strength seems gone,
But Grace lifts me up into His loving arms.

The day our youngest child was born, I learned to tread the water with both feet. I was afraid as they laid that beautiful, squirmy child on my stomach, and looked at her in disbelief. I couldn't process that she was here. I asked them to take her, to clean her off, and when they went to hand her to me again, I told them to give her to my husband.

It wasn't that I didn't want to hold her—I was terrified. Something in me figured something bad would happen if I touched her. I kept thinking—

What if she dies?

Sort of a weird thought to be thinking while your baby is inches away from you. She looked perfectly healthy, but I thought it nonetheless.

I held her later, but still refused to enjoy her. Being that vulnerable wasn't a reality where I could exist. I had done so well to keep myself together through natural childbirth, and I kept the same resolve on my face and in my heart.

My doctor was concerned about my 'lack' of emotion. She knew my history, of course, and the new baby and I stayed in the hospital together for four days instead of two or three. The doctor asked me was I ready to go home, and even though I was as nervous as a first time mom, I said yes.

I couldn't even figure out how to put her in the car seat. I started crying and one of the nurses helped us, and said not to worry about it.

My seventh child, and I couldn't even figure out how to put her in the seat.

I Didn't Miscarry Her...She Died.

She'd make cute little noises,
　　　　but I refused to acknowledge how cute they were.
　　　　　I had to keep it together.
　　I had to be a new mommy happy with her new daughter.

But inside my head, I still missed the child that would never be put in a car seat. Enjoying any moments with the new baby, seemed to BETRAY the mourning of the lost one.

It's quite a task, learning how to cry but not fall to pieces. Learning how to laugh, even though something in the new baby's steps reminds you of the little toes you won't ever see. I'm not sure it's something that is too complicated to explain, or if it's so simple it evades us below some invisible radar.

We are, after all, only human.
It's not an excuse, it's just reality.

We are so much harder on ourselves, than any person on the planet would be. I think motherhood includes a list of invisible rules that even though you don't see them, if you break one—everyone knows.

I Didn't Miscarry Her...She Died.

The number one hidden rule seems to be: Carry your child to term. Along with that, we must solemnly swear to insure no harm comes to that child before, during or after birth. (No pun intended on the after birth thing.)

So when any link in that chain gets bent, WE BECOME THE UNSPOKEN FAILURE, the woman who didn't have her healthy baby. No, no one ever says it to our faces, but their body language dictates their discomfort when we walk into a room.

Instead of embracing us and giving reassurance, people act awkward, as if we have the "lost a baby" plague.

No two people handle this the same way.

"When you reach the end of your rope, tie a knot in it and hang on."

—Thomas Jefferson

We've all met them. Those super women who seem to breeze through this type of loss, without even seeming to shed a tear. They go to work days after, call you as if nothing ever happened, and chalk it up to something that happens in nature.

Then, of course, there are those who don't consider a fetus a baby, so they have no idea why you're still upset. They consider your loss like a cyst being discarded, and can't for the life of them figure out why you're still remembering a due date of a child you lost years ago.

I used to feel like I needed to say something to people like that. It's almost like an attack, when people talk about how idiotic it is to name a child whose gender you weren't even sure of. People who smirk, who after learning you lost a baby that was never born, think you're being too dramatic or insane.

Well hooray for those of us who don't come unglued or need anyone else's help to deal with this type of loss. I hold no judgments toward anyone who feels like it is a thing of the past, which they can leave behind and not think about year after year. But I and so many like me couldn't get through the depth of this, WITHOUT GRABBING ONTO THE ROPE. I couldn't bear the literal pain that was created in my heart.

I Didn't Miscarry Her...She Died.

Most of all, I needed to know that I was loved and didn't deserve to hurt this way. I craved reassurance that the pain, though never gone, would dull and be a part of me. Some part of me that I could learn from and see with different eyes. I will never be the same type of mother I was before *Sarah* died.

Now, I hope I can be an even better one.

"So let me get this straight; _____ I can be happy, even though my baby died?"

Of course you should be happy! As miserable as you may feel sometimes, you don't deserve to be sad. *No matter what we feel we have ever done wrong or right in this situation, no one deserves to be held beneath the waters of sorrow.*

I'll always be thankful for my mother, reminding me about David in the Bible. He lost a child, too. The circumstances surrounding it were quite dramatic, and current day soap operas pale in comparison to this story. Whatever the catalyst, David and Bathsheba lost a child. People were astounded by his behavior.

He answered,
"While the child was still alive,
I fasted and wept.
I thought, 'Who knows?
The Lord may be gracious to me and
let the child live.' But now that he is dead,
why should I fast?
Can I bring him back again?
I will go to him,
but he will not return to me."
Then David comforted his wife
Bathsheba…
2 Samuel 12:22-24.

We can't be afraid to find out what it's like to be happy on the other side. Even though it's hard to see, there is an 'other side' to having lost a baby this way. Even when the sky is dark, light exist somewhere beyond it. A light that is so bright, that even when we close our eyes in death, it far outshines the passing of a soul from within us.

How does a person find the courage? It exists in the fiber of our skin, and in the substance of our souls. Survival is changed for me now. MORE THAN JUST EXISTING ON THE PLANET; IT IS TRULY UNDERSTANDING THAT MY EXISTENCE CONSIST OF OPTIMISM. I find myself thankful now, for things I may not have truly understood.

Courage is resistance to fear,
mastery of fear,
not absence of fear.

———————

Mark Twain

Pregnancy seemed to be something that just happened. Now I know it is not an entitled event.

It is a blessed event that not all will get to experience.

So each time, **every single time**, someone gets to announce that they are having a baby,
it is a miracle of wonder.

And for those of us who have experienced one or more losses, you don't have to carry the weight of the word *miscarriage.*

You didn't miscarry anything... your baby died.

It's ok to grieve, however you need to do that. I don't recall hearing about a book on the exact way you are supposed to grieve. Sure, there are people who tell you stages, but I skipped around all of them in the first day.

It took awhile,
    but I wrote her a note...

Dear Sarah,

Your life was but a glimmer, but it shone so brightly into mine. Your voice was never heard, but I hear you all the time. I never felt the softness of the hair upon your head, but one day I will touch the face, which means more than words have said.

My dearest Sarah you remain, the meaning of what is love, and I will lay my head beside you, when we meet above.

—Love, your mommy—

The holidays are the hardest. Her due date, well, you know.

The first Christmas that I hung seven stockings up, I felt the eighth one missing. I hesitated as I hung the last one, and I felt dizzy. I stood back looking at the wall, and felt my husband walk up behind me.

"Just hang one up for **her**," he said.

He already knew what I was thinking. I didn't hang one up with the other children's, but I brought a tiny Christmas stocking and put it on the tree.

Why?
It made me feel better.

I would never be buying her Christmas presents, or hear her squeal with laughter, when we put up a Christmas tree. But you know what I did do? I gave her a stocking. After I put it on the tree, I wrote her a letter.

My Dearest Sarah,

 If I could write the perfect letter to you today, what could it possibly contain to express what I feel in my heart for you? I don't know if I possess the skills with which to adequately relay what I know to be true. I miss you being here with us, but this year I want to smile so you will remember your Christmas watching me.

 I'd rather have you here in my arms, but until then, I have to believe you can see and know me from afar. I love you so much. All your brothers and sisters miss you. Daily they remind me of how I know you would be if you were here. But then again, you are here, aren't you, Sarah? I feel you watching from beside me sometimes, and I smile. I can't wait to see the reflection of my smile in your eyes when I see you.

 I love you, and I hope you are having a good time with Jesus today. Happy Birthday, Jesus! It is so good to know all of your Christmas Days will be spent in such bliss and love. It warms my heart to know that you will never know suffering and pain, only love. So today, I hope you see mommy smiling up at you, because I know you're smiling down on us.

 (((((((((((((Hugs)))))))))))))

I Didn't Miscarry Her...She Died.

I still have the letter, and I still mean every single word.

Some women might find comfort in other
children's voices, and I love all of my children,
but at first...the first year,
it was hard.

The past couple of Christmases,
I have found myself able to smile
and enjoy the sound of laughter.
I guess the phrase *'bitter sweet'* would be appropriate.

So I had to apologize.

On our youngest daughter's first birthday, I took her in my arms and inhaled deeply. Her sweet baby hair, in curls, smelled absolutely amazing, and she smiled up at me.

I cried as I apologized to her,
for being so afraid to love her.

I apologized for the nervousness I'm sure she felt,
every time she made a sound.

I apologized for not enjoying my pregnancy with her,
as much as I should have, even though I had done
the best I could at the time.

Something in me felt *free*, and the innocent look in her eyes confirmed what I always knew. No matter how I had been in the past, I loved this child with all my heart, and she knew it. Even though it was hard to relax, even though I can't really remember joyful moments during my pregnancy with her, I will forever be grateful to God for allowing her to be with me.

So what do I do when the due date rolls around?

Each year that passed, I tripped out on August 23rd. Some years I wouldn't even be thinking about it, and someone would say the date out loud, or I'd have to write it on a piece of paper. *All of a sudden, all of the loss would wash over me again.*

The strangest thing though, has to be the regulation of my monthly cycle. Even if I just had a period or wasn't due to have one for a week later, I always start one on the 23rd of August. I've been to therapy, even done hypnosis, but it remains. I literally have what feels like contractions, albeit not debilitating, and then start a period.

I'm sure if there are any psychiatrists reading this, there's some illusive diagnosis to be thrown my way, but I don't worry about it anymore. I'll be the first to admit, it's weird and perhaps unusual, but maybe someone else has this experience.

One year, a friend of mine said her ultrasound to find out the gender of her baby was on August 23rd. I didn't even think about it, and told her to let me know the results. She hesitated and then asked, "But is it going to upset you because it's on the twenty-third?"

First of all, *how amazing is that friend?* I couldn't believe she remembered, but she too knew what it was like to lose a baby this way. Secondly, I really hadn't thought about it. When she e-mailed later to say it was a girl, I took it as a sign.

Life really does go on after death.

You're born...you die.

I for one would rather celebrate the first occasion, but I learned to truly be happy for her on this day.

I Didn't Miscarry Her...She Died.

So now...I sometimes let pink balloons go,

and watch as they float away toward Heaven.

I sit and go through her box of things, trying desperately to remember her being within me. I may shed a couple of tears, but it's not overwhelming like the earlier years. Now, it's almost like my own little tribute service, where she can be acknowledged. Doesn't she deserve that much?

Sarah may not have been born into this world, but she was definitely birthed from my heart into the very consciousness of me.

She will always be a part of my experience.

Months go by and no one says her name, but as her mother, I always feel her. As time marches on and people forget about my seventh pregnancy, I couldn't forget if I tried. Some random cashier at a store will wear a nametag, that says *Sarah* on it and I'll think of her. I'll be watching a television show, and someone will call out her name. It's seems weird, but I've caught myself gasping.

I used to feel overwhelming sadness at these moments, until one night. I was crying myself to sleep, so sad and broken by the loss of my precious baby. I looked up toward the ceiling, and asked God just for one moment.

I needed one moment, to touch the face of my child and know that she was real.

I woke up in the middle of the night, aware that one of the children was standing beside my bed. Sleepy, I leaned up on one arm and said, "Rose?" I thought it was one of our other daughters. When the figure didn't move, a weird feeling overcame me, and I reached out. I distinctly felt the face of a child, but it was foreign and the height was all wrong.

Like a bolt of lightning, I sat up and could barely make out the dark silhouette of a child. I could feel the outline of a cheek and reached up further to touch her hair. It was unlike any of the children's hair that was in the house. Immediately, I called out, "*Sarah?*" INSTANTLY, THE FIGURE WAS GONE.

I jumped out of bed and turned the light on. I ran down the hall to our girls' room, and went up to each of their little beds. All three of them were fast asleep. I went into the boy's room, and my eldest son was asleep on the top bunk, while the twins were in their cribs fast asleep.

Walking silently back to my room, my heart was beating so fast. I knew, beyond a shadow of a doubt, that my Sarah had visited me. No one, and I mean no one, can make me believe otherwise. Through my fingertips, I could describe exactly what she looked like, and I know my eyes will see the child that I felt.

Page 101

Was it a psychotic episode? (Shrugging) I don't know, but if so, I'm grateful to have had one. I don't pretend to have all the answers about the afterlife, but I know what I felt and the shadow that I saw. Every day I am thankful for that little visit, because I know it was just for me. It was a message that it was ok to move forward, and somehow I had to allow myself to smile again.

Over the years, I've realized that *Sarah* wouldn't want me to be sad. I don't know what they do up there exactly, but I wouldn't want my child to see my crying every day. I want her to know how much she meant to me,

and that I choose to live for her.

THE EASTER BUNNY
HAS CLOSURE

---

*I always like to look on the
optimistic side of life,
But I am realistic enough to know
that life is a complex matter.*

———————

Walt Disney

Ok, so CLOSURE also tops my list of hated words in this world. When people started to see that I was doing better about my child dying, I heard tons of phrases that included this stupid idea. Maybe it works for some, but nothing was going to totally absolve my grief and

carry me to the magic land of happiness.

Oh, and I especially detested people using the word who hadn't even lost a puppy in life. You know, those educated relatives and friends who, just because they've taken psychology in college, figure they can asses you.

Better yet are the people who don't have or want children telling you how happy they are that you've "moved past" your obvious depression. I used to get aggravated, but eventually saw past their words and realized their ignorance. There was no way I would be able to explain to them, what took me years to be able to admit to myself.

Moving on I'm finding is prime,
But moving on took me a lot of time.
I haven't moved from missing her essence,
But I have moved from grief's effervescence.

Fake smiles from people, who don't remember my name,
Fake hugs from friends who aren't glad I came.
Fake responses from me that sounded sincere,
When, actually, I wanted to smack them in the ear.

Remembering the birthday of those alive,
Is it so different to remember one who has died?
After all the debate and all of the fuss,
A baby was growing, now there's just mistrust.

I don't trust myself to handle the tears,
Sometimes I'm afraid when things get too near.
But I want to be happy and embrace so many things,
Even though I'm distracted, by baby angel wings.

So when I think about her,
I know it's alright to daydream.

Every great dream begins with a dreamer.
Always remember, you have within you the
strength, the patience, and the passion
to reach for the stars to change the world.

Harriet Tubman
Activist

Now I have learned to appreciate
what I did have with *Sarah*.

I got to be excited about a positive pregnancy test,
many people don't.

I got to experience ten weeks of her beautiful spirit growing inside of me,
many people have never felt that.

And I was there, the moment her soul departed,

and I know she went from my womb straight into a different type of warmth.

It's comforting to know *Sarah* will never know pain or sorrow. She will never catch a cold, end up in the hospital, or have her heart broken when she starts dating.

She will only forever know happiness and utter joy.

But someone may ask, 'How are the dead raised?' With what kind of body will they come?
1 Corinthians 15:35

There are also heavenly bodies and there are earthly bodies; But the splendor of the heavenly bodies is one kind, And the splendor of the earthly bodies is another.
1 Corinthians 15:40

Will babies be babies in Heaven?

Ok, so once again, I'm just a mom, who has asked this question so many times, I stopped asking and started trying to figure it out. The only place I knew to look was the Bible. After all it had been the core of my beliefs for so many years, why not?

So why does it matter? *Do I really need to know that my baby went to Heaven?* Does anyone need to know that? I don't know. (Notice I say that a lot.) It's just something a mother wonders, when she doesn't even know what her child's face really looked like.

There are just some things I'm never going to know, and I've learned to accept that. There are all sorts of mysteries and things that my little mind could never comprehend.

But I found comfort in knowing that our heavenly bodies are different from our earthly ones.

It's going to be really great to look down, and not see stretch marks and cellulite. Even better, we won't even care about stuff like that. So, knowing whether or not my baby will be little or big, has become less of an obsession.

Now, I find comfort just knowing she will have a heavenly body and so will I.

A woman has so many gifts to bestow.
The delicate smile, that lies beneath her nose.
Hips that sway and will also bear,
Little, carbon copies her husband's heirs.

Upon a mother's death, the scene is very sad.
Husbands have died, children cried,
and her enemies aren't mad.
A trip to Paradise awaits, her body never the same,
Oh, the joy of knowing this, her weight will never change.

Arrival to this place I wonder, what will it be like?
Will I recognize my baby will she be a beam of light?
I find comfort knowing this, one thing I will not wonder,
My child will be in Heaven too,
my heart swells as it ponders.

Is it ok for me to think there's some type of baby, sitting angel, that sits with the spirit of my child and gives them hugs and kisses?

Ok, sure, the afterlife isn't exactly like this one, but it brings me comfort to believe my child isn't aimlessly floating around not knowing anyone.

I surround myself with <u>happy things.</u>

One of the best things I do now is surround myself with things that bring a smile to my face. After the initial shock of losing a baby, there are so many days full of tears and sorrow. And it's not the normal kind of tears you cry, it's the ugly kind that leave you messed up, with snot running all over your face.

Those tears end, and then you sometimes find yourself still sobbing, unable to put sound to the pain that you feel inside your heart. And let's not forget the physical aspects. I had downright contractions, and even though it lasted about five minutes, it was shocking to go through that and not have a baby in the end.

Now mind you, I went from one baby leaving my body, to another inhabiting my womb rather quickly. So to me, I felt like a piece of warmed over crud for an immeasurable amount of time.

It seemed like a marathon of torture,
designed especially for me.

And don't get me wrong, I am so thankful and fortunate that I was able to get pregnant so soon after losing *Sarah*.

I definitely believe, if I had not gotten pregnant with Sunshine, a part of my mind would have never returned. I look at her now, bugging her father who is trying to eat his dinner, and I am in awe.

I was blessed with this amazing little person,
even when my faith was small and weary.

Even when I was ticked off at God, I was blessed.

Yes That's What I Said. I had days I was so angry at Him. I didn't blame Him exactly, I was just angry that this became part of my life's story.

Once again, I know you know the super Christians. The ones who condemned me for being too sad, the ones that said, "God won't give you more than you can bear." I found most of those people had never lost a baby from the uterus, or had even had a child in the hospital.

They always wanted to remind me how they prayed for me, and while I valued prayer, the condescending ones probably never got higher than the ceiling anyway.

I'm singing a happy tune, even when I feel like crying. ——— ——— A.k.a. thinking yourself happy———

I was blessed to be able to play the piano at a young age. Music has truly been a comfort through all of this, and I sincerely believe we are given talents that can help us through the hard times. I wrote a song entitled '*Sarah*' that was instrumental only, and another song called 'This Year,' in memory of my dear friend David and *Sarah*.

The song that bears her name, I actually wrote just before my trip to the ER. Ironically, she is the only child I wrote a song for while she was in the womb.

I sincerely believe it was her gift to me.
It is a song without words that allows
me to recall her essence.

Some people sing, draw, do photography, write, etc. I found playing the piano, or blasting Frank Sinatra and dancing around to be great therapy. I've always been fascinated with King David in the Bible, and one of the reasons was because he was a musician.

When King Saul had an evil spirit upon him, David played the harp and it relieved him from his agony. It was definitely a gift that the Lord gave him, not only to renew his own spirit, but to comfort Saul. (1 Samuel Chapter 18)

So what is closure? Apparently, I think it's as imaginary as the Easter Bunny, but that's based on my experiences with people telling me I need to get some. I finally decided to make up my own state of being with it.

My closure entails:

crying when I need to,

being angry when I need to,

and being happy when I need to.

Some days I find myself really mad and angry.
I figure somehow my mind constantly blames me.
For the death of a baby I wanted to bad,
Now there are moments I'm angry...but also sad.

Some days I find myself feeling sad and alone.
I'm presumptuous enough to think I could
do this on my own.
Miserable days mount a perch and remind me,
There's no way I can just put all this behind me.

Some days I find myself searching around my mind.
I'm sitting still then I'm wondering,
'Will peace come in time?'
Will I one day awake and find I'm not in so much pain?
Even Sunshine comes after a tornado and rain.

Some days I wake up, and before I step out of bed.
I think of the things I'm thankful for...instead.
Instead of sorrow and guilt flying around,
I'm thankful for peace that exists within the sounds.

I'll never shut the door on this experience, because it's part of me. To act as if I never lost a baby would be absurd. But, I am learning how to exist within the sea of ups and downs. I'm learning to accept myself as human, and realize that I am doing the best I can.

I don't have to apologize for my humanity,
I need to realize it and accept love to compensate.

You gain strength, courage, and confidence by every experience by which you really stop to look fear in the face.

PRAYERS AND PAIN, FORGIVENESS AND RAIN

You are able to say to yourself,

'I lived through this horror.
I can take the next thing that comes along.'

Eleanor Roosevelt

I'm sure we all have a list of people who have done horrible things to us in the past. We may or may not have acknowledged the issues, forgiven them and moved on. But the forgiveness that I'm talking about doesn't have to do with anyone else.

It has to do with forgiving yourself.

You know that place that was feeling guilty for the loss of your child? Well, I found that I blamed myself for so long that loving myself was near impossible. If you don't love yourself, how can you be the best wife, mother, daughter, sister, or woman you can be?

How many times have we not cried out for help, because inwardly we didn't feel we deserved it? And even though you might say you know it wasn't your fault the baby died, we still have moments of thinking we could have changed the outcome.

We are only human,
we cannot change the past;

however, that doesn't stop us from thinking over the entire pregnancy, wondering what we could have done different.

Understandably, there are some who feel their activity caused the demise of their child. Drug use, smoking, drinking and other factors as such have been known to cause harm to a baby. But what about women who do all those things and have healthy babies? Some people drink or smoke up until the day their child is born, and end up having perfectly fine deliveries and babies.

So what does that mean for those of us who didn't do those things? People who took prenatal vitamins, and ate healthily, exercised moderately and chemically had nothing that attributed to the demise of our children?

There's no simple answer, and even if there were one, does that bring back our children? Sadly, no. Forgiving yourself doesn't have to do with admitting guilt or a mistake, it means letting go of the responsibility you feel that wasn't in your control. So if anything, you're forgiving the ignorant part of yourself that blames itself for something it had no control over.

So I try to see
          through the tears,
but it's hard.

No one wants to be sad, but you can understand your sadness. We are all so hard on ourselves, and expect perfection on so many levels. We feel that we disappointed everyone by losing the baby, and we are exceptionally hard on ourselves. *If it were one of your friends that had lost a child, what would you say?*

We have to become our own friend. Be kind enough to yourself, to lean on other people. Those tears can be heavy, when they are yours alone to bear.

People can be a resource for you,
to strengthen you and
help you see the joy that exists in your life.

One of my biggest questions all the time was...

How do I get my *joy* and p e a c e back?

I was looking for that one simple thing, that if I did it, I would be back to the self I knew before the loss. Well, unfortunately, I found out that 'one thing,' does not exist. There is no magic potion, no immediate thing, that makes all the pain go away and you're like you were before.

In America, we live in a society of quick fixes. Most people are looking for that faster, easier, quicker thing that makes life the way they want it to be. But to expect something so grievous, to be resolved quickly, isn't realistic.

Can you imagine childbirth with no pain?! That would be AWESOME, right? Breezing through nine months, and then in the end, having this wonderful birth that doesn't even hurt. Ahhhh, how wonderful would that be! But is it realistic? Of course not!

We find ourselves moaning, screaming, panting, or anything else that gets us through the delivery. And even though we go through all of that isn't it amazing how we find ourselves wanting to do it all over again? Why, because the end result is worth every pain.

So I started thinking. Losing a baby, as devastating as it is, doesn't have to deter our desire or reality of getting pregnant again and truly enjoying the process. I was so focused on my loss, that during my next pregnancy, I couldn't really be present and cherish every milestone with the new baby. I wasn't truly giving thanks at the time, because I was too immersed in guilt, pain, sadness and fear.

Even though I didn't have the right tools when I first lost *Sarah*, I have them now.

Now, I can miss her and be a better mom to my living children. Now, I could get pregnant and enjoy every moment, and know that it doesn't lessen my love for my lost child.

A baby growing in my belly, wow,
I wish that could be true.
To feel the joy I've felt before,
and know there was life anew.
A blessing from God, if it should happen,
I'd take it as a sign.
That life goes on despite the sorrow,
and happiness can be mine.

Oh, God, how I'd give anything
to hear a heartbeat from inside.
I'd tell every soul I ran into I don't
think anyone could hide.
To know that life within you grows,
no greater gift I know,
I just keep praying every day,
the Bible tells me so.

I'm not entitled, that's not what I feel,
as I ask God for this.
I just want one more little face,
to smell to smile at, to kiss.
It's in my soul every moment I wake,
before I go to sleep.
"Dear God, please bless me one more time,
with tiny little feet."

So many people think I'm nuts, surely,
she must have lost her mind.
But they don't know what I now do;
children aren't promised, all the time.
Every time someone gets to announce,
"A new baby will be born."
It is a blessing for that woman,
with nurturing she is adorned.

Another baby...yeah, ok, I'll admit it.

Even though most people I know will think it is nuts, I would love to have another baby. I'm a few years older sure, and the medical community loves to give you scary statistics. But at this rate, if I listened to statistics, I would have never gotten married and had over two children.

I believe that a woman can know in her heart, if she is meant to be a *mother*. Some people dream of being doctors or television journalists, but I've always wanted to be a mother. And though I have a houseful of them running around even now, I always feel like there is another little person that should be here.

I'd be remiss to say that all women should experience this, because some don't want to. I don't believe it makes them alien to our gender,

I believe it's their right of choice.

After all, God is pro-choice. _____

"But if serving the Lord seems undesirable to you,
then choose for yourselves this day
whom you will serve."
Joshua 24:15

Pretty simple concept. We can make choices in life that will either make us happy or sad. I believe we all have a Devine right to be happy. That's hard to do if you don't forgive, love and accept yourself and your body.

If we can really believe that God is pro-choice, it doesn't mean He gives us an excuse to do the things we know are wrong. This is not a statement made lightly with the intent, that people should be allowed to do things that they believe are wrong. Nor is it an excuse to hurt others.

We need to make informed and wise choices. Hopefully, we will make choices that allow love to shine through us.

Knowing that we have a choice brings a sense of relief.

Can you believe that if you want to be happy and find peace, all you have to do is choose it? It seems so simple, but many of us struggle with allowing ourselves permission to believe this.

It is your choice.

The uneven circle of life is crazy.

SO HERE'S THE GOOD NEWS.

Nothing Devine made your baby die, it died.
People are born, people die.

Part of pregnancy involves the fact that sometimes things go wrong. Sometimes chemicals in our bodies or hormones are off. Sometimes there is no reason given for the demise of a baby.

It does seem extremely out of order anytime children die, because people are intended to grow old gracefully. Of course it's terrible, whether it be through childbirth or a car accident, homicide or natural disaster. A child dying before their parents is one of the most difficult things to handle.

Losing your baby provides an opportunity to strengthen your faith. Believe me, it took awhile for me to want to accept that. I kept thinking,

"My baby was allowed to die, and I somehow deserved it."

What I'm learning is, thinking that way makes me feel more guilt and remorse. But both those things didn't have to become my crosses to bear. No one was meant to suffer, and holding on to that disables me as a woman. My self esteem suffered, and my ability to love and be loved was basically non-existent. Love doesn't feel guilty. Guilt and love couldn't exist in the same place.

We can learn from every situation that occurs in our lives. I am learning so many things about my faith that I would have never sought out, if I had not lost *Sarah*. Would I rather have her here running around? Yes, but I can't control that. I can only control my resolve and perseverance.

Page 129

When love leads you, there is no _____ confusion.

There is always the danger that we may just do the work for the sake of the work.
This is where the respect and the love and the devotion come in—
That we do it to God, to Christ, and that's why we try to do it as beautifully as possible.
_____

Mother Teresa

Wanting another baby is sometimes so prevalent to women that they will go about it in various ways. People can become desperate in their quest. Some people, whether married or not, figure the quickest route is the best route, and that's not the best criteria to go by.

Praying about every decision you make is an awesome opportunity to see miracles in life._____

The Vatican is against surrogate mothers. Good thing they didn't have that rule when Jesus was born.
Elayne Boosler

There is always a debate about single women having artificial insemination, or having a pregnancy come about the old fashion way and keeping the child. There are debates about couples undergoing in-vetro fertilization, or using a surrogate to grow their child. Whatever choice people make, ultimately, is between them and their creator. Children are a blessing, but I don't think you can acquire them, with a 'by any means necessary' mode of thinking. That being said, you do have the right, to do anything that is ethically within your means to do. There is no obstacle that a mother wouldn't climb for her child, even if it hasn't been born yet.

We hold these truths to be self-evident: that all men are created equal; that they are endowed by their Creator with certain unalienable rights; that among these are life, liberty, and the pursuit of happiness.
Thomas Jefferson

Not everyone will support the choice That you feel is _____
_____right for you.

Someone who claims to be your best friend can say the most unsupportive and hurtful things. Do you want to smack them? **Sure**, but don't. Family members are going to tell you how crazy you are, and sometimes they can be the worst. That is why praying about your choices, and knowing what you truly desire, is paramount.

No matter how you feel you need to procreate, pray. Pour out your heart and admit all that you desire. Allowing oneself to be vulnerable to this desire is the best way set yourself free to acquire it.

If you want one baby, say one. If you want twenty, say twenty. If you want as many as you can have, all you have to do is ask. I found this really cool story in the Bible.

In bitterness of soul Hannah wept much and prayed to the Lord. And she made a vow, saying, "Oh Lord, Almighty, If you will only look upon your servant's misery and remember me, and not forget your servant but give her a son, then I will give him to the Lord for all the days of his life."
1 Samuel 1:11

And here's one of the coolest things in the next few verses.

> As she kept on praying to the Lord, Eli observed her mouth. Hannah was praying in her heart, and her lips were moving but her voice was not heard. Eli thought she was drunk and said to her, "How long will you keep on getting drunk? Get rid of your wine." "Not so, my lord," Hannah replied, "I am a woman who is deeply troubled. I have not been drinking wine or beer; I was pouring out my soul to the Lord."
> 1 Samuel 1:12-15

Even the priest looked on her actions and misread them! Here was Hannah broken hearted, pouring her soul out, and someone assumed something about it. All she wanted was a son. She went to the Source, to get an answer, and was judged harshly for that choice.

Church. When I was first going through losing *Sarah*, church was the worst place. So many people said the wrong things at the wrong times, not guided by God, but by their own opinion on my situation. You have to be very careful of people who tell you things about and from God, just because they are Christians.

Having the title of a *Believer of God*, does not automatically mean someone has quality advice. A month after I lost *Sarah*, I walked into a church so down-hearted and sad. I actually had someone walk up to me and say, "Hey, at least you have...hmm, let's see, (they counted my children) six children. You should be happy with that."

I Didn't Miscarry Her...She Died.

Of course I was thankful for my six children,
but my baby had just died.

Give me a break!

What kind of supportive statement was that?
So if their child had gotten hit by a car, would they have
liked it if I had said the same thing?

Not everyone will have a baby.

Ok, so it had to be said.

Not everyone will give birth. No matter how much you cry and pray on your knees, you may never endure the length of labor you desire. Your labor will be much different. You may labor with the disappointment of never getting pregnant, or having multiple losses from the womb.

No one can foresee what will happen on this journey, and therein lays the foundation of fear. The fear of not being able to just get pregnant and have a healthy baby, can resonate and shatter our hearts. This isn't said to be a discouragement, it just ends up being some people's reality in this life.

But I didn't need to hear that, while I was mourning the loss of my daughter. No one needs to hear that! What I needed to hear was that no matter what, my family and friends would be there for me. I needed to know that even if they thought it was insane, they would support what I felt in my heart. We should all be allowed to pursue this desire,

unashamed and with vigor.

I Didn't Miscarry Her...She Died.

Some people say that losing a child that has lived with you, is worse than a pregnancy loss.

Here is a debate that should not be debated. People want to qualify loss, and make women, who are sad about a miscarriage, feel that they are not entitled to have the same sense of sadness. Well, who made them judge?!

I am thankful that I have not lost a child outside of my womb. I am truly sorry and compassionate to those parents who have lost children to sickness, accidents, homicide and more. But I will not apologize or say that their pain is greater than mine, because they have more memories. I will not say that my pain is greater, because I don't have the cherished memories and life time experiences. **That's the point.** We shouldn't be arguing whether the sadness is justified. Anyone who tries to console you by saying, "Well, at least you lost it early on," is ignorant to what you are going through.

Does gestational age determine the amount of sadness you feel? No.

Should someone miss a four year old murdered child, less than they miss a child who was twelve?" No.

Those questions have the same answer. Accept that some people just aren't going to get it, and don't get hung up on the details.

You don't have to justify your grief, no more than you would if your sibling or parent died.

It is not length of life,

but depth of life.

_____

Ralph Waldo Emerson

DON'T WORRY...
BE A MOTHER

I walk slowly,

but

I

never

walk

backward.

Abraham Lincoln

That title seems a bit odd, but it can be true for you. Think about it this way. You are only human.

You are only one person.

How can one person expect to carry around all that you deal with as a woman, and then add on top of that losing a child and wanting to have another?

It's even crazier when you have other little children running around. Not only are you trying to deal with this issue, you're trying to take care of the emotional and physical needs of little people who need you.

And if you don't have other children making life interesting, you may have a job or environment that literally has you overwhelmed enough. How can you expect yourself to deal with all this by yourself? Would you expect the same thing out of a daughter?

Of course not.

The most amazing resource for us...*LOVE*.

It is never ending, and abundant.

Love wouldn't leave you anxious and nervous about having a baby. Sure, the whole childbirth part bites, but after the contractions are over, your life is so full you forget about them.

Losing a baby from your womb is sort of like that.

Yes, it hurts.
Yes you are in pain you have never felt before,
or that you never wanted to feel again.
But the pain eventually lessens.

No one sprints around a day after giving birth and expects herself to fit in the clothes they wore before pregnancy. So why would you expect that of yourself after losing a child?

You CAN NOT expect your body or your spirit
to be exactly like it was before. But the cool thing is...

You don't have to do this alone.

Even when some people have forgotten about your loss, and don't want to validate the pain you are still in, someone will rise out of the ashes and be there for you. Sometimes the pain can be so debilitating, that we forget to ask for help. But it's not only important to ask for help, we must go to a good source for it. I felt like sometimes I set myself up for stupid comments to be made. You know, you try to talk about how you feel to people who don't have more sense than your dog.

And Lord knows why I was a repeat offender some days. Maybe, I thought if I could just explain it right, these people would understand where I was coming from. It's so important to assess the character and intentions of people, when seeking advice or support. When you are dealing with a loss where you are already in such a vulnerable state, you have to be careful.

The wrong comment can make you cry for weeks, and end up undoing months of progress.

Four Tips:

Don't expect your SINGLE friend.
who doesn't want kids.
to comfort you.

**Don't talk to relatives who don't think
you need to have another baby.**

*Don't listen to doctors who
only want to tell you outcomes
and not possibilities.*

**Don't expect negative people
to have positive things to say.**

(That last one is a Godsend.)

Page 144

I had a friend who told me,
a child will come in time.
She sat rocking two of her kids,
but consoled me to wait for mine.
I had a friend, who told me,
just pray and give it to God,
I prayed every day, but I'd have to say,
that didn't do the job.

I had a friend who told me,
it must not be in His Will.
But she's been trying in-vetro,
more times with doctor's skills.
I had a friend who asked me,
why do you need anymore?
I guess if I had to explain,
on our friendship I shut the door.

A relative thought their advice,
was witty and very sound.
They treated their children horribly,
and liked when they weren't around.
Another one thought their advice,
would make me feel way better,
I'd rather they had kept to themselves,
my eyes only got wetter.

So now I've learned that some conversations,
I never should have had.
Why in the world would they say such things,
knowing I was already sad?
People are ignorant, and some plain dumb,
I'm sure you know it's true.
So I decided to surround myself,
with women who want to be mothers too.

I Didn't Miscarry Her...She Died.

All of those situations can set up
an environment of depression.

NO ONE NEEDS TO BE DEPRESSED,

and if you're excited about eventually having a child, don't
let anyone take that excitement from you. You owe it to
your future children to be the happiest mommy you can
be. That includes while they are in your womb,

or while you're signing adoption papers.

Uh, oh, I used the...

'A' word. _____

Ok...adoption. Some people are just not down with it. Once again, that is completely their choice. But why not? Yes, having a baby growing inside of you is amazing. Yes, pregnancy is an awesome experience that I for one love and would love to do again.

But what's so bad about adoption?

It doesn't mean you've failed. It means you've opened yourself up to having children, however you can. There are hundreds of children all over the world, praying daily that they could have a mommy. They pray the same prayer as you, except reversed.

Your uterus might be jacked up,
your tubes or other plumbing might be shut down.
Your husband might not have enough swimmers,
or he had a bike accident when he was twelve.
You may not be able to physically have children because of
some genetic issue,
or disease that you have.
Some people have heart issues,
blood pressure,
chronic diabetes etc.
Are they less qualified to be mothers?
Of course not!
One of the ways you hear the sound of children's laughter,
may be through adoption.

Being a mother brings happiness.

Anything can happen. I think sometimes we get so hurt and disappointed we stop believing or give up hope.

You have to have **hope**, in order to have children.

So much goes into having a baby or adopting a child, and if you lost your faith, you would crumble through both processes at some point.

Go ahead, I dare you...believe.

If patience is worth anything,
it must endure to the end of time.
And a living faith will last in the
midst of the blackest storm.
Mohandas Gandhi

What would happen if you really believed you could have a child? What if you had to believe it for a year…two… three? Does it mean enough to you, that you would still hope for ten years, without worrying about when? Well, if you said yes, you're probably better off than me.

It literally terrifies me to think about waiting for anything. I think it is part of human nature to want things immediately. If there were a way to commit to the idea, wouldn't it be great just to believe it, and be open to any opportunity that would provide?

Now, or course, you can't just sit around hoping for something and not doing anything about it. I believe we were commanded to be fruitful and multiply, and given a really cool way to accomplish that. (Ok, for those of you who just blushed, I'm sorry, but it really is cool.)

So, it won't work out if you wait for a baby to fall from the sky. You've got to have faith, but you also have to do something about it. Believing is an action word. Assuming that whatever happens, happens, sounds sort of ridiculous. The fact that you want a child is one thing—you also have to believe in what you want. So much so that every fiber of your being cries out and proclaims the desire of your heart.

I found new characteristics of faith.

All who call on God in true faith,
earnestly from the heart,
Will certainly be heard,
and will receive what they
have asked and desired.

———————————

Martin Luther

There were so many days I was barely holding on. People had no idea that I felt like I would snap at any moment. Telling me to just have faith, implied that I didn't have any. If they only knew, that it took every ounce of faith to get out of bed.

Faith to believe something bad
wouldn't happen to my other children.
Faith to believe my heart wouldn't fail me.

You are doing the best you can, and you are still here. We have faith that people could never understand, even if they tried. There is no substitution for falling into the ashes of faith that is born of the fire of grief. It rages faster and more furious than anything you could ever know. It suffocates you, but keeps you alive long after the flames die down.

So my faith was still there, just singed around the edges.

> You do because you are.
> You can because you love.

You can live through losing a baby. You can live through the struggle of trying to become pregnant. You can be happy if you get pregnant again, and you can overcome the fear of another loss enough to try.

Everything that you need to be successful and happy can be found. Search for answers, pray and ask those who have walked down this path for help. Many of us receive just as much in return if we can share what has supported us throughout the days, months and years. Nothing happens by accident. You don't have this book in your hand by accident.

You are a **strong**, beautiful woman. You have been through something that has hurt you, more than anything you could imagine. We will always bear the scars of this labor, inside our hearts and some physically. *You are not alone.* Many of us are familiar with the pain, although each story is different and the outcomes varied.

Consider yourself VALIDATED.
Your ticket has
been
officially
—————————————————stamped. –

If I had a major point of this book, it would have to be VALIDATION. You lost a baby or possibly many babies. There was no dropping the ball, or mismanaging as the word miscarriage implies.

I personally know women who have been planning a nursery for years, and several times thought the crib wouldn't be empty...but it is. Some have gone on to have children, several more in some cases, but they still remember the baby that never took a step.

No one can decide how this chapter goes on for you. Only you have the power to choose.

Isn't that the great thing?
You actually can control something...
your **actions** and **attitude**.

Certain thoughts are prayers.

There are moments when,
whatever be the attitude of the body;

the soul is on its knees.

————————

Victor Hugo

I Didn't Miscarry Her...She Died.

I want to say something that makes it okay,
I want to give in to what I feel...stay in bed today.
But I've got to survive this and somehow go on,
If I don't make it, then how will her name go on?

Somebody give me some place I can fall,
Some place I can admit, I've lost it all.
Let me scream let me holler, let me feel all the pain,
Let me fight against the darkness, the best way I can.

If you tell me it is ok then maybe I'll believe,
I can't hurt anymore than this, what is it to be me?
Can you see the way I feel; will you say it is ok?
Please, give me a moment and realize I'm hurting today.

So, I'm going to get up and go...keep fighting going on,
My baby died...wow; I can't believe I just typed that.

A positive attitude does wonders. —

Even bound up in adversity, you can acknowledge the good in life. There are others who support you, find them. Associate with people who share the same desires and outlook, and you will find the encouragement you seek.

Line up all advice and support with what you truly believe, and you will be amazed how blessed you will be. Not only with the hope of having children, but with more knowledge about who you are as a person.

Will you be perfect? uh...nope. Will you get pregnant immediately after reading this? Maybe. (Smile) But most importantly, hopefully, you have a few more tools to support you on this path.

Many of us have mothers who watch us deal with these issues. I thought it would be neat to add some thoughts from my own mother, Grace D. Myers.

First is a letter that she wrote me.

I Didn't Miscarry Her...She Died.

My Dear Daughter,

    I heard and saw you crying in your room today, so much pain and heartbreak, no words could I say. My first thought was simple. "Lord, why couldn't it be me?" You've suffered through so many things and this just was not fair! It made me look to heaven and ask, "God, don't you care?"

    Then I said, "Forgive me, Lord, You care for us each day." Michelle, I'm at a loss for words, it seemed the thing to say. And yes, I said those words again, throughout this sad, sad day.

    Would you want to hear me say, "It's alright and ok?" My generation always spoke these words, "it just happens sometimes this way." Then I think how stupid that sounds, you won't hear that today.

    So, I'm asking Jesus. "Lord, what would you have me to say, to give my daughter comfort in her lost today?" And not just for your loss alone...for my grandchild went away.

    God's words were gently spoken to my heart this day, and my loving daughter, His Words to you I'll say. In time your heart will strengthen, take all the time to cry. For His Grace is sufficient and His love is no lie.

    Yes, your heart is broken, His heart is broken too, and He knows the loss you feel...He lost a child like you. Just take each day one at a time, find comfort in all that's true. For one day up in Heaven, they'll be no night or past. There with Baby **Sarah**, you'll be at peace at last.

                                  Love Mom

Silence

One day your heart was broken
Lost words were never spoken.
In silence I could pray
Lord, help my child today.

And though there are no words
To mend the hurt inside
I watch you strongly hold your own
Each day to just get by

Some days are harder than others
Expected as should be
But let my love shine through your pain
And may you always see
You'll never suffer things alone,
For you're always a part of me.

Mom

PLEASE, JUST SHUT-UP

I've learned that people will forget what you SAID,

people will forget what you DID,

But people will NEVER forget how you made them *feel.*

Maya Angelou

I Didn't Miscarry Her...She Died.

This road is not an easy one to travel, and some days, it's made all the worse by words people say. Sometimes, the best intended words miss the mark. Sometimes, it would have been better if nothing were said at all.

Over the years, people have said some real interesting things to me about losing my baby. I'm sure you have your own, or know someone who does. I'm a true believer, in knowledge being power, and *ignorance being the fuel for folly*. So maybe if the following things were mentioned aloud, women who suffer this type of loss wouldn't have to endure the outcome of well intended remarks.

Things NOT To Say
When a Woman Has Lost a Baby
_____ during Pregnancy _____

1. God will bless you one day.
Reason: This one implies that God isn't blessing her now.

Alternative: I know it might not seem like it, but God knows your hurt and loves you.

2. It wasn't really a baby yet, you don't have to be so upset.
Reason: Are you kidding me? This one should be apparent if the person is completely falling apart. Of course they acknowledged the child growing inside of them.

Alternative: I don't understand what you're going through; I've never lost a baby while pregnant.

3. Weeping is only for a night, joy comes in the morning.
Reason: Gee, thanks for sharing a scripture, but being a sparkle of sunshine isn't always best. When someone is grieving, you have to give them time to be sad. People grieve in their own way, in their own time.

Alternative: If you need to talk, I'm here. I might not always understand, but I'll listen.

4. At least you have other children. Focus on what you have and not what you don't posses.
Reason: You're saying she shouldn't be sad about her child dying. That's stupid. If your child died, would you want someone to say that to you?

Alternative: What can I do to help you with the other children?

5. You're young enough to try again.
Reason: You're implying she can just replace the baby that died.

Alternative: I'm sorry for your loss.

6. Sometimes these things just happen.
Reason: Sounds good, but this one reinforces the fear that bad things can happen at any time. If she gets pregnant again, thinking that something can 'just happen,' is a constant thought.

Alternative: No matter what has happened or will happen, I will be here for you.

7. Have you thought about adoption?
Reason: Sounds like you're confirming that her attempt at having a baby has failed. It's better to let her bring up the idea.

Alternative: I know you want to be a mother. Anything that I can do to support you, I will.

8. I didn't even know you wanted a baby.
Reason: Makes it sound like you don't think she should be upset.

> Alternative: I know this was unexpected, I'm sure this isn't easy for you.

9. I lost a baby once, and it didn't upset me at all.
Reason: You sound like a jerk. Everyone handles this differently.

> Alternative: I lost my child once, I'm so sorry you're going through this. We all deal with it differently.

10. Maybe it just wasn't the right time to have a baby.
Reason: Once again, you sound like a jerk. Who made you the judge of someone's life?

> Alternative: I don't know why this happened, and I'm sorry you're hurting. I'll be here for you.

11. Oh, my sister's friend's cousin's uncle's friend's grandma's niece, lost a baby once. She got pregnant again real soon.
Reason: Nobody cares and it's not a personal connection. And the last thing someone wants to hear; is about someone else getting pregnant soon after their loss.

> Alternative: I haven't personally lost a child, but I know someone who has.

12. I put you on the prayer list at my church.
Reason: Thanks, but that also means you've probably told people I lost my baby. It's not your place to tell. If you are going to put me on a prayer list, just mention my name and don't tell me.

> Alternative: I'm asking God to be with you in this hard time. You have many people who pray for you and we love you.

13. Are you going to "so and so's" baby shower?
Reason: You've either forgotten, or are brushing aside the fact that it might be difficult for her to go to someone else's baby shower. It's inconsiderate.

> Alternative: Don't ask!

14. Maybe being around babies will help you feel better.
Reason: "May bees don't fly in September." You have no idea if it will help or not.

> Alternative: Don't suggest it!

15. Are you going to try again?
Reason: It's none of your business.

> Alternative: Just shut up.

16. You are older now, things tend to happen as you age.
Reason: Thanks for the vote of confidence. You've basically told the woman she's too old to have a healthy pregnancy and baby. Most times, an older mother is more educated about her physical state. There's no need to remind her.

Alternative: Sarah had a baby at over a hundred years old. Go for it! (Of course only if you know this person really well.) If not, just give them a hug.

17. You still look pregnant.
Reason: Obviously she may assault you.

Alternative: Don't mention it.

18. You can have one of my kids, they're terrible.
Reason: You sound insensitive, even if you do really mean it. If she's trying to get pregnant and have a baby, your offer is an insult.

Alternative: You're going to be an amazing mother. You're so good with my children.

19. I've got some information on how to up your odds on not having a miscarriage.
Reason: It implies she didn't do her best to avoid one the first time around.

> Alternative: I don't know if you want to talk about it, but I've got some interesting things I found about losing a baby.

20. What did your husband say?
Reason: He might have been relieved, or been a total idiot about the entire thing. He might have cried for days and needed depression medication. Either way, it's none of your business, even if you are a relative.

> Alternative: We're praying for your entire family.

——————— Resources ———————

Ok, so I was pretty mental when this all first started. *I wasn't sure where to look or what to do.* Having a computer was really cool because you can Google just about anything. The sites that helped me the most are listed below. I really did go to them, and I really did find good information or support.

As with most things, I don't fully support or know every detail about any of these sites. I mention them solely because of their informational content.

About.com Pregnancy & Childbirth
    http://pregnancy.about.com/
American Pregnancy Association
    www.americanpregnancy.org
BabyCenter   www.babycenter.com
    www.pregnancy.com
BabySnark   www.babysnark.com
CafeMom   www.cafemom.com
Christian Mom   www.christianmom.com
Medline Plus   www.medlineplus.gov
Merriam-Webster Online   www.merriam-webster.com
Pregnancy Center WebMD   www.webmd.com/baby
Pregnancy.org   www.pregnancy.org
Womenshealth   www.womenshealth.gov
Michelle's Website   www.michelle25.com

For those who are struggling with emotional issues, such as DEPRESSION or ANXIETY, I encourage you to seek the care of your healthcare professional. I have found some wonderful doctors in my area, but it took a great deal of searching and investigating.

Take the time you need,
pray and choose wisely.

Remember, just because someone went to medical school and has a license doesn't mean they are right. Get a second opinion, a third opinion, and talk to other women. Some of my best resources were from other women who had experienced loss or were having fertility issues.

Medication for any reason during this journey does not mean you are a weak person. *It means you're strong enough to recognize when you need assistance, in being the best person you can be.* Natural remedies have also been amazing for me, and it can never hurt to have a healthy diet and good exercise routine.

Meditation and prayer works wonders on the body. Take time to nurture yourself, and love the body that was created for you. I pray you are blessed as you travel this path.

And remember, you didn't miscarry anything...

your baby died.

By three methods
we may learn wisdom:
> First, by reflection,
> which is NOBLEST;
> Second, by imitation,
> which is EASIEST;
> And third by experience,
> which is the BITTEREST.

————————

Confucius

I Didn't Miscarry Her...She Died.

————— Acknowledgements —————

My mother, *Grace D. Myers*, for always supporting my dreams and taking care of my dog, when I left and went to college. For being there, when I was a complete mess, and helping me to stand.

My husband, RON C. WALTERS, for pursuing those dreams with me and being an amazing singer/songwriter. Without you, there is no music; a life without song is no existence at all.

My *seven beautiful children*, for saving me from myself and allowing me to play in your fast paced world.

My brother, S. CHRISTOPHER PHILLIPS, for always being there for me.

My brother, MARK MYERS, for our younger years together.

Aunt Cathy Hawkins & UNCLE CHARLES, for your encouragement.

Donna Davis, for your greatest gift... Ron.

Carolyn Terry, for raising David to love the Lord.

Linda Ralls, for allowing me to find my voice in writing, and teaching me to never settle for "no."

Linda Brown, for encouraging me to push myself beyond the limits of my expectations.

DR. JOHN PITTMAN, for your resolve, to make things as they should be.

ROBERT SMITH, for tapping into my life and changing it.

Dr. Julie Morrow, for being a wonderful part of our village.

Acknowledgements

LaDonna Heintzelman, for **Sarah's** box of memories.

Christina Lawson, there's not enough room on the page.

Ashley Cavin Thomas, for having "a listening," and love.

JoEllen Poindexter, for understanding and comfort.

DR. CHUCK EDGINGTON, Ph.D., for allowing God to let you think outside the box and into our circle.

TRACY DECKER, *Carmen Sanchez*, JAMES BARTLETT, *Debbie Bivins McGlohon*, *Darla Calvird*, ROBERT PAIGE

DeAnne Dooley, for the peanut butter and jelly sandwich the day I completely fell apart in the workroom.

Kelly Danz Harrod, who took the time to ask how I was doing while going through something insurmountable herself.

Katie Fry, for listening, even when you didn't have time.

To everyone at Woolstrum Publishing/ Adsum Press
ANTHONY WOOLSTRUM, for listening to my rambling.
My Editor, *Kristen Woolstrum*, for believing in the work.
Publishing Representative, *Natalie Farr*

The wonderful staff of TODAY'S THERAPY SOLUTIONS

THE CONGREGATION AT NORTHWEST CHRISTIAN CENTER, for reminding me of God's love in the darkness.

In loving memory of my father,
MICHAEL R. MYERS & my friend CHRISTOPHER DAVID TERRY; who walk beside still waters with my **Sarah**, in the presence of our Lord and Savior, Jesus.

CPSIA information can be obtained at www.ICGtesting.com
Printed in the USA
BVOW04s0006090114

341363BV00013B/323/P

9 780982 014165